Alzheimer's and Dementia - Facts, Myths and Misconceptions

The Complete Beginner's Guide for Caregivers

Charles Seaton

Table of Contents

Introduction

The first thing that a person must understand, for caregivers especially, is that: dementia is not Alzheimer's disease, nor is Alzheimer's disease the same as dementia.

Dementia is a general word that is used to describe a group or set of signs and symptoms that can be caused by several disorders or conditions that involve the brain. People who suffer from dementia are observed to be not mentally fit enough to do everyday activities such as eating, getting, dressed, working, taking a bath, or even shaving. Because the brain is affected, they may lose some or most of their problem solving ability and skill. Part of the experience that they undergo includes slight changes in personality, loss of control over their emotions, forgetfulness, memory loss, and some agitation or anxiety caused by seeing their environment as unfamiliar.

Alzheimer's on the other hand, is just one of the diseases that might lead dementia. It is a progressive disease whose signs and symptoms include those that affect a person's memory, thinking, and behaviour. In simpler terms, Alzheimer's disease is a cause, while dementia is the effect. It is important to note however, that Alzheimer's disease is not the only cause of dementia; it is merely the most common one.

Most of the difficulties experienced by caregivers concerning patients with dementia and Alzheimer's disease are influenced by the numerous myths and fallacies surrounding the conditions. How the patients are perceived is colored by these opinions which results in misunderstandings and assumptions that might not benefit the patient or might cause outright harm to them.

Caring is the primary job of a caregiver; it is the root of the whole profession. One must understand that caring does not merely mean passively providing what is physically needed nor is it just following instructions on what to do. On a deeper level caring is about developing relationships and a sense of kinship with patents and clients. These relationships are the vehicles for therapeutic care that is holistically beneficial for all parties involved.

The one trait that makes a caregiver truly great is the ability to empathize. In order to give effective care, first know how you want to be treated yourself: think of the whole situation and try to put yourself in the metaphorical shoes of a person suffering from dementia.

In order for a dedicated caregiver to do all of that, it is important to dispel all kinds of judgements from the preconceived notions that are formed by the public misconceptions about Alzheimer's disease and dementia. Before anything else, get informed. Know the facts and the truths behind every concept of care: know who you are caring for, what to expect, how to treat them, and the significance of how long term care can help.

The contents of this book will hopefully serve as a guide to most of the things that you need to know and be prepared for as a caregiver for sufferers of Alzheimer's disease and dementia. Read on and take the very first steps to learning and caring.

Chapter 1:

Who are These People?

Myth 1: Dementia is an "old person's disease."
Related Myth: Dementia is a natural part of the aging process.

The Facts:

Dementia is a medical condition and is not an inevitable occurrence that comes with age. Old age may be a risk factor but not all who reach mature ages eventually acquire dementia. While it is true that most cases of dementia sufferers are reported to be of the elderly group, it is not exclusively confined to them only. Depending on the cause which could sometimes be head injuries, substance abuse, stroke, or infections, dementia can happen to people as young as thirty years old.

Aside from age, other risk factors that influence the occurrence of dementia and Alzheimer's include sex, family history, and heredity. Those who have family members who have suffered from dementia have a slight genetic predisposition to eventually developing the same condition. Statistically, there are higher rates of dementia among women than in men.

Characteristics of People with Dementia

People suffering from Alzheimer's disease and dementia have the one or more of following problems:

- memory loss
- reduced thinking abilities and thinking speed
- some impairment in speech, language, and communication
- altered ability of understanding and judgement

People who have dementia can become passive or completely apathetic about their previously usual daily activities. They may have some trouble in controlling their emotions and may have various behavioral changes that are very different from how they were before. At times, they may find social situations awkward and difficult. For some, they might even lose interest in the whole process of socialization. Other characteristics include:

- loss of empathy and compassion
- some hallucinations or delusions
- planning and organising difficulties
- depression
- changes in both personality and mood
- Periods of confusion

Chapter 2:

Normal and Abnormal Behaviors: What to Expect

Myth 2: People with Alzheimer's disease or dementia act violently and are generally aggressive.

The Facts: Not everyone who suffers from dementia or Alzheimer's disease become aggressive. The disease affects every individual differently and their reactions to these effects vary as well. The memory loss that comes with dementia can be very frustrating for a lot of people and some might even find it frightening. The frustration, fear, and anxiety might sometimes be manifested in acts that might be perceived by others as violent.

Myth 2: People suffering from Alzheimer's disease are unable to understand what is going on around them.

The Facts: While dementia can cause some confusion, this does not immediately mean that the person does not know what is happening around them; they just might be having some difficulties. As the disease affects mental abilities, the process of making sense of things might be slower but it does not affect a person's intelligence. Assuming that people with dementia cannot understand things can lead to alienation due to hurt feelings. A person afflicted with dementia is still the same person he was and is no way less smart, less observant, and less understanding of his surroundings.

Myth 3: Dementia sufferers either don't know what they want or are unable to communicate exactly what it is that they want.

The Facts: Most people who suffer from dementia know what they want but have some trouble with the communication part. As a tip for caregivers, it is sometimes helpful to take note about patterns in behavior to determine the like and dislikes of the patient. In this case, when verbal communication becomes difficult, reading body language is an important skill to develop.

Myth 4: People with dementia do not know or are not aware that they have it.

The Facts: During the early stages of the disease, it is not uncommon for a lot of people that something might be a little bit off about their memory and cognition. They may notice that they are having some slight trouble completing usual tasks. This awareness however declines as they progress through the later stages of dementia.

Behavioral Issues of People with Dementia

There are certain behavioral changes that can occur as a consequence of the effects of dementia. Although this varies form case to case, most of the sufferers of dementia feel so many negative emotions: anxiety, fear, confusion, frustration, and even sometimes a feeling of being lost. Each individual deals with these emotions in his or her own way. Some of the most common behavioral manifestations of these feelings include:

- Repetitive questioning and/ or activities
- Pacing or continuously walking to and fro
- Shouting, screaming, and other acts of aggression
- Some paranoia or lesser form of suspicion of other people

How to Cope with Behavioral Changes and Problems

As caregivers for people who exhibit these kinds of behavior, it is important to keep in mind that these are done in attempts to communicate something. It is not always the case that patients with dementia are deliberately trying to be stubborn or difficult. The key to being an effective carer is to keep calm and patiently try to work out the reasons behind the seemingly odd behavior.

If you are able to recognize patterns in behaviour and certain warning signs that may come before an outburst, escalation of any situation may be prevented or avoided.

1. **Repetitive questioning and/ or activities**: These are ways that some people with dementia deal with loss of memory, anxiety, boredom, or pent up excess energy. In some cases, it may be a side effect of medications.

How to Cope: If the behavior is out of boredom then think of a good activity to distract or engage them with. Some good suggestions are listening to music, art activities, or simple games. Actions done out of anxiety can be lessened when patients feel that they are reassured and supported.

2. **Walking continuously or pacing back and forth**: Pacing is quite common among people with dementia but this is usually a phase that will resolve itself after a period of time. The reasons why they walk repeatedly and continuously have various reasons, some of which are: forgetting where they originally intended to go (maybe a shop or to visit a close friend); out of boredom or a desire to get out of the house for a little exercise; or confusion about times and places they should be in.

    How to Cope: One of the main concerns when people with dementia tend to wander is the possibility of them getting lost and being unable to find their way back. This can be avoided by letting people concerned know about the person's condition. An identification bracelet can be worn by the patient with pertinent contact numbers. There are also some types of assisted technology devices that can be employed to help track them down in case they get lost from walking. The best suggestion to avoid any unnecessary incidents is to accompany the patient while he or she walks and gently assist them whenever they feel lost.

3. **Aggressive behavior and violent actions**: People suffering from dementia may occasionally show signs of aggression as a result of

the following causes: fear, humiliation, frustration, and depression, impairment of judgement, loss of inhibition, or loss of self control. The most common forms of aggressive behavior are: shouting, screaming, use of offensive language, and repetitive calling out for something or someone.

How to Cope: The best way to avoid aggression is to try to pinpoint triggers that may cause the behavior. It is important not to aggravate the patient by arguing or by dealing with them in an aggressive way as well. The aggressive actions stem from the illness and are rarely personal or intentional.

4. **Suspicion of others**: This is usually due to some memory loss, confusion about the state they are in, and lack of recognition of anything that is familiar.

   How to cope: Because people suffering from dementia are unsure of a lot of things, situations, and people this makes them seem a bit delusional or paranoid. It is important for a caregiver to remember that these fears or feelings are not completely unfounded and are very real for the patient. Listening and calming them down through distraction or subtle changing of subjects can help.

Chapter 3:

To Do or Not to Do: That is the Question

Myth 5: Correcting a person with dementia is the right thing to do when he or she does or says something wrong.

The Facts: It is best to not correct a person with dementia when he or she says something that is not quite right. Constantly correcting the person can lead to several negative results: alienation from the patient, depression, combativeness and aggressive behavior, and further confusion. It is important to note that he or she has lost some memories, some ability to think clearly, and some reasoning ability. All of these results to the irregularities or inconsistencies of the things that they say.

The Best Ways to Help:

- Be sensitive about what they perceive as failures or shortcomings
- Try to avoid being overly critical of their attempts
- Offer support and gently offer any help when it is badly needed
- Use memory aids or visual signs to help them remember where important things are
- Promote independence as much as it is prudent to allow without endangering the personal safety of all people involved in the care.

Myth 6: People with dementia and Alzheimer's disease are incompetent.

The Facts: This myth does not apply to all people who suffer from Alzheimer's or dementia; it is dependent on how far gone the stage of dementia is. In the early stages of the disease, people are fully capable of making decisions and functioning normally. Care during the later stages would be most beneficial when a balance between independence and reliance is struck.

The Best Ways to Help:

1. **Hobbies and Interests**: Many people with dementia are still capable of enjoying hobbies and interests such as cooking, painting, drawing, running, dancing, singing, listening to music, or gardening. Depending on their interests, they can be enlisted to perform chores or tasks that would help to make them feel useful around the household or around people they interact with in a group.

2. **Incontinence**: This can be caused by a number of things such as urinary tract infections, medications, outside pressure on the urinary bladder, or the patient with dementia simply forgetting to go to the toilet in time. It could also happen that he or she has forgotten where the toilet is or is unable to communicate his or her need of going to the bathroom to the caregiver. Whatever the

reason, the experience of incontinence can be a very upsetting situation for any person. The best ways to deal with this are:

- Have a sense of humor to keep from embarrassing the patient further
- Put clear and understandable signs on toilet or bathroom doors
- Make sure that the toilet is easily accessible to the patient with dementia
- Help the patient when he or she experiences difficulty in taking off clothes due to zippers, buttons, or snaps.
- Be alert for signs that the patient might need to go to the bathroom
- Make use of incontinence pads, adult diapers, or waterproof and rubber beddings.

3. **Good Health and Nutrition**: Staying fit and being healthy physically can contribute to the quality of life that they lead. Having little nutrition can lead to susceptibility to other illnesses, diseases, and infections. Most of the issues about food and eating are caused by confusions or some minor delusions that they might harbor due to the effects of dementia. Some of the common problems one might encounter are:

   - not recognising the normal foods or meals set out for them to eat
   - forgetting what kinds of food they prefer, like, or don't like

- refusing to be fed or spitting out food they don't feel like eating

- resisting attempts of being fed

- asking for strange food combinations or imaginary food stuffs

The main point to remember is to involve the patient so he or she does not feel forced into changing eating habits. In time, he or she can adjust to new arrangements and schedules. It just takes a little patience to keep both caregiver and patient less stressed about meal times. Taking the patient's old and new food preferences into consideration will help to encourage him or her to eat and enjoy the meals that are prepared for him or her. Some special considerations that need to be discussed among family members of people with dementia and healthcare providers are smoking, drug use, and alcohol consumption. It is of course best to avoid these habits but if the patient has had them for a long time, some issues about withdrawal symptoms may arise which could make them more confused and anxious.

4. **Personal Hygiene**: Some problems that a caregiver might encounter include:

- Safety issues: there is always the risk of slipping on wet surfaces and falling, especially when the patient feels disoriented or dizzy.

- Privacy or lack of it: Some patients may be uncomfortable washing or bathing themselves when somebody else is around, even if there is an intention to help.

- Refusal to be helped or uncooperative patients: This is most often due to extreme embarrassment or stubbornness and a feeling that they can do personal things by themselves.

When helping a person with dementia to perform activities for personal hygiene, the essential thing is to be quick and efficient to avoid any unnecessary exposure of skin and any undue embarrassment. Privacy is also big issue that should be taken into consideration. When a patient prefers a close relative or loved one present, it also helps to ease some discomfort. Safety measures are of course always to be taken to avoid accidents and injury. Rubber mats or rugs can be strategically placed to avoid slippage and some support bars may be installed for the patient to grip on while getting in and out of a tub or shower. Make sure that the patient is within earshot and easy reach distance when he or she does any task by himself or herself.

5. **Sleep and Rest**: There are cases when patients with dementia can have trouble sleeping. They can wake up in the middle of the night or feel too restless to sleep. Problems like this usually tend to get worse as the dementia progresses to its later stages. A caregiver can take some measures to ensure a good night's rest for the patient. Sleep improvement methods include:

- Limiting naps during the day
- Avoiding consumption of coffee, tea, cola, and sugary drinks at least four hours before bed
- Setting a schedule to establish good sleeping patterns

Caring for People with Dementia

Having dementia provokes a lot of negative emotions and feelings for the person suffering from it. They are most likely to feel anxious, stressed, and even frightened. The awareness of the increasing deterioration of their memory paired with some physical clumsiness can lead to frustrations and feelings of helplessness.

Caregivers can make their clients or patients feel more secure by creating an environment where they feel relaxed and are encouraged instead of criticized. Giving them a regular and consistent routine can help them feel more empowered and more able to face the stresses of performing everyday activities.

Encouraging some independence and allowing them to do small, uncomplicated tasks or chores can help to make them feel more confident and useful. This contributes greatly to their self worth and self esteem. As the illness progresses and independence versus reliance becomes a bigger issue, more support and patience will be needed for their care.

Ways of Encouraging Communication

- Remember to speak as clearly and as slowly as possible. A good tip is to use short and simple sentences that are easy to understand.

- Face the person and make eye contact when appropriate.

- Pauses and moments of silence are okay; sometimes it is best to not expect them to respond too quickly as they may feel pressured if they are rushed to give an immediate answer.

- Try to encourage the person with dementia to join in on conversations with others people when it is possible.

- Do not speak on behalf of the person with dementia during important discussions on their personal health issues. This can take away their independence and make them feel invisible and might result in them not speaking up for themselves anymore in other conversational situations.

- Provide simple choices and avoid complex sentences that might cause confusion.

- Do not ridicule or criticize answers that might be off topic or inappropriate.

Communication is one of the keys that might help to make the whole caring process successful. In order to be aware of the needs and preferences of the patient, clear communication channels must first be established for the benefit of all parties involved. As much as possible, persons with dementia or Alzheimer's disease are encouraged to verbalize, so as to get them to socialize and at the same time keep everything clear and understandable.

Be fair in assumptions and judgements; although it is best not to make any in the first place, there are some instances that they cannot be avoided. As a caregiver for people with dementia and Alzheimer's disease, it is important to keep these assumptions at a bare minimum. Do not let judgements color your capacity to care. People with dementia are still living. Breathing, human beings and as such deserve to be treated well, despite of their unfortunate luck to be stricken with a condition that makes them less than adequate to engage in proper communication with people around them.

Caring for Your Own Wellbeing

As the primary caregiver of a person with dementia, it is just as important to maintain your overall wellbeing as it is to help the patient achieve his or hers. The job of caring can be extremely frustrating, stressful and tiring. When it gets to a certain point or limit, taking a break or resting can help to dispel the tension. A healthy and happy caregiver means a healthier and happier patient as well.

Chapter 4:

The Miracle Cure All for Alzheimer's and Dementia

Myth 7: Dietary supplements can protect the brain. They can help to prevent, and treat Alzheimer's and dementia in general.

The Facts: There are no strong evidences to support the claims that vitamin supplementation and other alternative methods can effectively prevent or treat dementia and Alzheimer's disease. Most are based on assumptions and possible theories that relate nutrients or chemical compounds to the inner workings of the disease processes involving the progress of dementia.

Can coconut oil help to prevent dementia?

As of the moment, there are no concrete evidences or proofs that coconut oil can either treat or prevent dementia. There are however some studies that aim to find out if some components of coconut oil can be potentially beneficial for dementia sufferers. The results concerning the research on coconut compounds and dementia have been so far inconclusive.

Are statins effective in lowering risks for dementia?

It is not recommended to take any supplementation of statins as recent trials and studies have shown that they are not effective or successful in preventing Alzheimer's disease and other forms of dementia.

Is hormone replacement therapy a helpful risk prevention method?

It is generally not advised or recommended for anyone to start hormone replacement therapy as a means of dementia prevention. The studies that concentrate on finding a link between Alzheimer's disease and hormone replacement therapy have mixed and confusing results: some show that hormone replacement therapy increases the risk of dementia while others suggest the opposite. More research on the matter is needed for a more conclusive and reliable answer.

Is aspirin good for a patient with Alzheimer's?

Non-steroidal anti-inflammatory drugs, otherwise known as NSAIDS and which includes aspirin, ibuprofen, and paracetamol are being explored as drugs that can possibly reduce the risk of developing Alzheimer's disease. At the moment however, studies have not yet been fully completed and clinical trials are yet to be done. It is not advisable and recommended for a person to take such drugs as preventative measures against Alzheimer's disease until the completed studies about their benefits are put out for the public.

Should I recommend the following for people with dementia?

B Vitamins: Taking in vitamin B supplementation will not prevent Alzheimer's disease or dementia. It might be helpful in improving the thinking skills of people with high levels of homocysteine in their body. But it cannot improve the cognition abilities in elderly people. Evidence of its benefits has to be studied well before anybody can be completely sure of its abilities related to dementia and Alzheimer's disease.

Gingko Biloba: Gingko biloba is not effective in slowing down the progression of the disease processes involved in dementia and is likewise not effective as a prevention measure for the disease. It does was shown by studies to have no effect in improving thinking skills and the quality of life of people with dementia.

Caffeine and Ginseng: There are studies that have some suggestion of the benefits of caffeine and ginseng extracts that might possibly help in Alzheimer's disease treatment. The results of these studies however are mixed so further research into the matter many be needed before any firm conclusions are to be proclaimed.

Green Tea and Cinnamon: There are no known evidences that green tea or cinnamon have preventative properties against dementia. They are no concrete proofs that they can treat dementia or any of its signs and symptoms.

Side Note: Is there a connection between aluminum and Alzheimer's?
There is an ongoing myth that promotes cooking with aluminum pots or pans and using aluminum foil can increase the risk of developing Alzheimer's disease and eventually dementia. This was proven to be a fallacy; studies have failed to bring out any conclusive evidence to attest to its truth. Most scientists and experts of the medical filed have agreed that exposure to the normal sources of aluminum in the environment does not contribute to the threat of dementia development.

Myth 8: Alzheimer's disease is curable.

The Facts:

Even with the current advances in modern medicine, there is no cure for Alzheimer's disease. Treatment is mainly focused on ways that slow down its progression and development; even then, medication only slows down the worsening of signs and symptoms by an average of six to twelve months. The methods and techniques of dementia treatment are done to help people suffering from it to live independently for as long as possible and to live a better quality life for the remaining years allotted to them.

For the Caregiver:

A caregiver should be aware about issues concerning the many "cures" and "treatments" that many people are willing to try just to get better. It may help to be informed when the chance pops up that the patient or family members of the patient may ask some questions. Understandably, wanting to get cured is something that they would desire. It is important to be supportive and hopeful while at the same time realistic as well to prevent wastage of any valuable resource and effort.

Chapter 5:

The Sad Truth about Alzheimer's and Dementia

Myth 9: Alzheimer's disease is not fatal.

The Facts: The sad truth is that Alzheimer's disease is a degenerative condition. It can be fatal as a result of the destruction of well needed brain cells. Memory loss also includes the body forgetting the functions it needs to perform to sustain life. The abilities to talk, move, and eat can be forgotten which makes it difficult for the physical body to survive. Dementia in itself on the other hand, is not fatal; memory loss does not directly cause death although the after effects might lead to accidents or injuries that might pose a possible threat on a person's life.

Myth 10: There is no hope for people diagnosed with Alzheimer's disease or dementia; there is nothing good about being diagnosed with the disease.

The Facts: Although there is yet a permanent cure for Alzheimer's disease, researchers and experts are still continuously finding better ways to detect and diagnose the disease, better ways of treating it, and even finding ways of developing a vaccine. There is still great effort and resources put into the whole learning process about Alzheimer's disease, its treatments, and management methods that aim to lessen the effects of symptoms and improve the quality of life in general. A diagnosis of

Alzheimer's disease or dementia does not mean the end of the world or the end of a person's life. As long as there are people to provide good care and adequate support, dementia sufferers can and will live a meaningful life.

Although being diagnosed with Alzheimer's disease can be very devastating news, there is always a silver lining to every dark and ominous cloud. In a sense, a crisis like this can strengthen bonds between families, patients, and the group of caregivers and health workers who are all involved in care. It is a testament to the strength of people and the tenacity that keeps everyone going. It is a situation that involves a lot of trust, patience, understanding, and kindness. On one hand, dementia and Alzheimer's disease can be viewed as tragedies that strike unfortunate people. On the other, it can be seen as a catalyst that brings about extraordinary change in people who would have not otherwise realized potentials of caring without the occurrence of sickness, illness, or disease.

Conclusion

The one important thing we can take away from the whole learning process of caring for people with dementia is that all people deserve to be treated well with dignity, respect, and patience. Being aware of what one might face when dealing with patients will prepare you for the tasking but fulfilling job of caring for them and their families as well.

Study, learn, and grow from the experience then pay it forward; share the knowledge and continue to give hope to Alzheimer's or dementia patients and their families. Help everybody take the difficult but necessary baby steps of being aware and fully knowledgeable about the disease.

Part of caring is helping to educate the masses about the real facts of dementia and Alzheimer's disease, how to cope with it, and ultimately how to live with having such a condition or how to live with someone suffering from it.

Help to put an end to all the untruths, myths, fallacies, and misconceptions surrounding Alzheimer's disease and dementia: get the facts and learn about the disease process and effects of the condition; seek help through the proper channels when appropriate; and lastly treat all people suffering from the disease with utmost respect.